Reclaiming Homo Erectus:

The Self-Chiropractic Healing Guide to Upright Living

By: John Mercola

Contents

Disclaimer

The information provided in this book is intended for general knowledge and informational purposes only. It is not intended to be a substitute for professional medical advice, diagnosis, or treatment.

The content within this book is based on historical, anecdotal, and scientific research, and while efforts have been made to ensure accuracy, medical knowledge and understanding are constantly evolving.

Readers are strongly advised to consult with qualified healthcare professionals, such as physicians, oncologists, or other medical experts, before making any decisions or embarking on any treatment plans related to cancer or any other medical condition.

Every individual's medical situation is unique, and treatment decisions should be made in collaboration with a healthcare provider who can take into account the specific medical history, current health status, and individual needs of the patient.

The author and publisher of this book are not liable for any adverse effects or consequences resulting from the use of the information provided within this book.

Readers are encouraged to exercise critical judgment and discretion when considering any alternative or complementary treatment approaches discussed in this book.

This book serves as a starting point for understanding the potential benefits of natural therapies in cancer treatment, but it is not a substitute for professional medical advice.

Reclaiming Homo Erectus:

<u>The Self-Chiropractic Healing Guide to Upright Living</u>

Hippocrates, Avicenna (سينا ابن), and Maimonides (ميمون بن موسى) put capital importance to the skeleton and the spine state. Both came from different religion and culture (Ancient Greece, Muslim, Jewish), but all agree on one truth that the state of spine is of importance for the health of the human body. They intuitively knew that energy flows past through the spine. This modern medicine ignores the spine and its state in health and diseases.

Avicenna in the Canon of medicine does not miss one disease or organ to treat without fixing and curing subluxation or deviation of the vertebrae to re-establish the current to the organ which is in agony acting like a flickering bulb waiting for the constant current to come to ignite it. They did this before Dr Palmer created the school of chiropractic medicine or Dr Still created the osteopathy.

You cannot cure or heal mechanical problems by chemical drugs. If the verterbrae T9 or T10 are out of orders, you cannot cure liver troubles by pills or supplement, because the supplement the current is not there. You are beating a dead horse.

Self-chiropractic healing is a unique approach to spinal health that empowers individuals to take control of their well-being by practicing self-adjustment techniques. This DIY method focuses on healing and aligning your own vertebrae, relieving subluxations, and correcting posture without the need for expensive professional chiropractic sessions. The beauty of self-chiropractic healing lies in its accessibility—it's suitable for both kids and adults.

Through a set of safe and easy-to-follow exercises, individuals can embark on a journey of self-care, promoting not only spine health but also enhancing overall vitality and well-being.

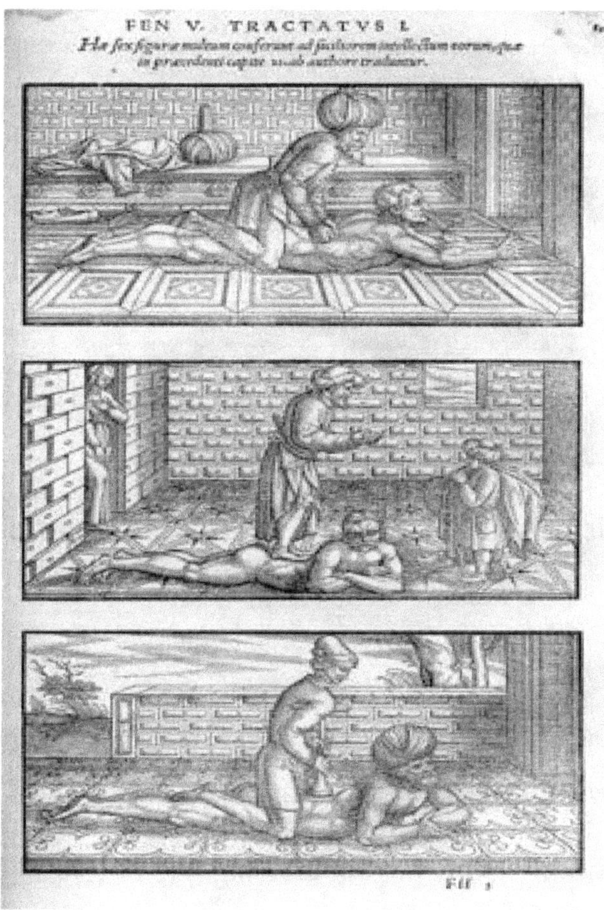

Understanding Self-Chiropractic Healing

Chiropractic care is a well-established field of alternative medicine that primarily deals with the diagnosis and treatment of mechanical disorders of the musculoskeletal system, particularly the spine. Traditional chiropractic care typically involves manual adjustments performed by trained professionals. However, self-chiropractic healing offers an alternative path, allowing individuals to engage in spinal adjustments independently. The essence of self-chiropractic healing revolves around the belief that the human body has an innate ability to heal and maintain itself when properly aligned. By applying gentle and controlled techniques, individuals can stimulate this innate healing power, addressing minor spinal issues and improving their overall health and vitality.

The Principles of Self-Chiropractic Healing

Self-chiropractic healing is built upon several fundamental principles that guide its practice:

Alignment: The central focus of self-chiropractic healing is the alignment of the spine. Proper spinal alignment is essential for overall health, as it ensures that the nervous system can function optimally, transmitting vital signals between the brain and the body.

Subluxation Relief: Subluxations, which are misalignments of the vertebrae, can lead to discomfort and pain. Self-chiropractic healing aims to relieve subluxations through gentle manipulation techniques.

Posture Correction: Poor posture can contribute to various health problems, including musculoskeletal pain and reduced mobility. Self-chiropractic healing exercises are designed to correct posture issues, promoting better spinal health.

Empowerment: Self-chiropractic healing empowers individuals to take an active role in their health and well-being. By learning and applying these techniques, individuals can reduce their reliance on costly professional chiropractic treatments.

Safe and Easy-to-Perform Exercises

One of the key features of self-chiropractic healing is its simplicity. The exercises involved are safe and can be performed with ease. When done consistently, these exercises can yield significant benefits for spinal health and overall vitality.
Let's explore some of the key self-chiropractic healing exercises:

Spinal Stretching: Gentle stretching exercises help improve spinal flexibility and relieve tension. These exercises often involve bending and twisting motions that target different areas of the spine.

Posture Awareness: Becoming aware of your posture is the first step in correcting it. Self-chiropractic healing emphasizes the importance of maintaining proper posture during daily activities.

Breathing Techniques: Proper breathing techniques can aid in relaxation and improve spinal alignment. Deep breathing exercises can be incorporated into your self-chiropractic healing routine.

<u>Mobilization Movements</u>: These movements involve controlled rotations and stretches that promote spinal mobility. They can be particularly helpful for relieving stiffness and discomfort.

<u>Self-Massage</u>: Gentle massage techniques can release tension in the muscles surrounding the spine, further enhancing spinal health.

<u>Progressive Relaxation</u>: Stress can have a significant impact on spinal health. Self-chiropractic healing often includes relaxation exercises to reduce stress and muscle tension.

<u>Visualization</u>: Visualization techniques can be used to mentally focus on the alignment and health of the spine, promoting a mind-body connection.

The Benefits of Self-Chiropractic Healing

Engaging in self-chiropractic healing exercises on a daily basis can bring about a wide range of benefits:

Improved Spinal Health: The primary goal of self-chiropractic healing is to enhance spinal health. By addressing misalignments and subluxations, individuals can experience reduced pain and improved mobility.

Better Posture: Correcting posture issues can lead to increased comfort and reduced strain on the spine. Improved posture can also enhance confidence and overall well-being.

Stress Reduction: Many self-chiropractic healing exercises incorporate relaxation techniques, which can help reduce stress and promote a sense of calm.

Increased Vitality: A well-aligned spine and reduced muscle tension can lead to increased energy levels and overall vitality.

Cost Savings: One of the most significant advantages of self-chiropractic healing is the potential for cost savings. By learning to perform these techniques independently, individuals can reduce their reliance on professional chiropractic care.

Empowerment: Self-chiropractic healing empowers individuals to take an active role in their health and well-being. It encourages a sense of self-reliance and personal responsibility for one's health.

Safety Precautions

While self-chiropractic healing can offer numerous benefits, it's crucial to approach it with care and responsibility. Safety should always be the top priority. Here are some important safety precautions to keep in mind when practicing self-chiropractic healing:

Consultation: Before beginning any self-chiropractic healing routine, it's advisable to consult with a qualified healthcare provider, particularly if you have any underlying medical conditions or concerns about spinal health.

Self-Assessment: Understand your body's limitations and listen to your body. If an exercise or adjustment causes pain or discomfort beyond a mild stretching sensation, discontinue it and seek professional advice.

Consistency: Consistency is key to seeing benefits from self-chiropractic healing. However, overdoing it can lead to strain or injury. Start slowly and gradually increase the intensity and duration of your exercises.

Proper Technique: Ensure you are using proper technique for each exercise. Poor form can lead to unintended consequences or injury.

Know When to Seek Professional Help: Self-chiropractic healing is not a substitute for professional chiropractic care. If you have severe or persistent spinal issues, it's essential to seek the guidance of a licensed chiropractor or healthcare provider.

<u>Disclaimer</u>: A prominent disclaimer should be included in any materials related to self-chiropractic healing, emphasizing that the information is for educational purposes only and not a replacement for professional medical advice.

Incorporating Self-Chiropractic Healing into Daily Life

To make the most of self-chiropractic healing, it's important to incorporate it into your daily routine. Here's how you can integrate these practices into your life:

<u>Morning Routine</u>: Start your day with a few minutes of self-chiropractic healing exercises to align your spine and promote good posture.

<u>Desk or Office Work</u>: If you have a desk job, take short breaks to perform stretching or posture correction exercises throughout the day.

<u>Evening Relaxation</u>: Wind down in the evening with relaxation and breathing exercises to relieve stress and tension.

<u>Consistency</u>: Consistency is key to experiencing the benefits of self-chiropractic healing. Make it a daily habit, and over time, you'll notice positive changes in your spinal health and overall well-being.

<u>Regular Check-Ins</u>: Periodically assess your progress and make adjustments to your routine as needed. Consult with a healthcare provider if you have any concerns or questions.

<u>Lifestyle Support</u>: Complement your self-chiropractic healing routine with a healthy lifestyle that includes a balanced diet, regular exercise, and adequate sleep.

<u>THE IMPORTANCE OF THE SPINE HEALTH</u>

<u>The human spine is truly the tree of life :</u>

The spinal column consists of a total of 33 vertebral bones, nine of which are fused together at the lower end to form the sacrum and coccyx. These vertebrae are arranged in a stack, resembling building blocks, and are separated by intervertebral discs made of cartilage. Each individual vertebra has a prominent oval-shaped bony structure known as the vertebral body. Additionally, there is a substantial opening at the rear part of the vertebra, situated behind the vertebral body, which is referred to as the spinal canal. Within this spinal canal, the spinal cord and nerves run, extending from the brain down to the tailbone. These nerves serve as the communication pathways, transmitting signals from the brain to the muscles and the rest of the body.

The robust sections of the vertebrae that form the sides of the spinal canal are called pedicles, while the sturdy bone that makes up the posterior part of the spinal canal is known as the lamina. You can feel a bony projection extending from the lamina when you touch your back, and this is called the spinous process.

Each vertebra forms connections with its neighboring vertebra through three distinct joints: an intervertebral disc and two facet joints. The facet joints are situated toward the rear of the spine on each side, in proximity to the lamina. The intricate interplay among these three joints at every level of the spine not only grants the spine significant flexibility but also ensures stability and guards against injury.

The intervertebral disc, a pliable cartilage cushion, possesses a dual-layer structure. Its inner core is referred to as the nucleus pulposus, while its outer, tougher layer is known as the annulus fibrosis. This disc serves as a shock absorber, facilitating spinal movement and flexibility.

On the other hand, the facet joints are compact synovial joints positioned at the posterior aspect of the spine on both sides, where they connect in the vicinity of the lamina. These facet joints are encased in a robust outer joint capsule.

The uppermost section of the spine is referred to as the cervical spine, and it consists of a total of 7 vertebrae. With the exception of the first and second cervical vertebrae, each vertebra at this level features three joints—a front-facing intervertebral disc and two rear-facing facet joints. The cervical spine is exceptionally flexible, which also makes it more susceptible to injuries. Additionally, the cervical spine has small openings on either side to accommodate a specialized blood vessel known as the vertebral artery, responsible for carrying blood to the brain.

Moving to the middle portion of the spine, we encounter the thoracic spine, which comprises 12 vertebrae. These thoracic vertebrae are intricately connected to the ribs and the breastbone, known as the sternum. The thoracic spine, due to its limited range of motion and flexibility, is notably robust and tends to be resistant to injuries.

Descending further down the spinal column, we arrive at the lumbar spine, consisting of 5 vertebrae. In the lumbar region, there is a significant range of motion in terms of flexion and extension, although rotation is comparatively limited. These lumbar vertebrae, being the largest in the spine, bear the brunt of the body's weight and endure substantial loads and stresses. It is unsurprising, then, that the lumbar spine is the most commonly afflicted region of the spinal column.

The lowest segment of the spine, firmly linked to the pelvis, is known as the sacrum. Comprising 5 fused bones, the sacrum forms a stable foundation for the spine. Furthermore, the coccyx, composed of 4 small bones fused together, constitutes the tailbone, marking the lowest extremity of the spinal column.

A vertebral subluxation, as described by the founders of chiropractic, D.D. Palmer and B.J. Palmer, refers to a condition where there is pressure on nerves, resulting in abnormal functioning and potentially causing a disturbance in some part of the body, either in its function or structure. It's important to note that subluxations may not always be discernible through X-ray imaging.

Chiropractors who adhere to the traditional teachings of Palmer continue to emphasize the significance of vertebral subluxation, contending that it can have a substantial impact on one's health. They also incorporate a visceral component into this definition.

The upright posture of humans, with a bipedal stance on their legs, offers a significant advantage by freeing up the upper limbs from the demands of locomotion. This liberation allows the hands to be utilized for both creating and using tools. This unique advantage, coupled with the cognitive capabilities of Homo sapiens, has been instrumental in granting humans intellectual and technological superiority over other species and creatures.

However, this advantageous posture also comes with its own set of challenges. The human body, when standing erect, places considerable stress on the spine due to the weight of various organs and the head. Any incorrect lifting or movement can strain the vertebrae, potentially leading to subluxation—a condition where the vertebrae become misaligned.

When subluxation occurs, there is a risk of these misaligned vertebrae pinching the nerves that pass through the openings, known as foramen, between adjacent vertebrae.

It's important to understand that nerves function akin to electric wires—they require freedom from compression or pinching to operate optimally. Even slight pressure on nerves can impede their ability to transmit signals effectively.

This interference can extend to the nerves' control over organs and blood vessels in various parts of the body, which can ultimately lead to health issues and diseases stemming from poor spinal posture or vertebral subluxation.

Many human ailments can be traced back to spinal deformities and subluxations. The specific diseases that manifest often depend on the location of these vertebral subluxations. Among them, cervical and dorsal subluxations are particularly concerning, as they have the potential to completely disrupt the functioning of the vagus nerve—a crucial component for relaxation and healing.

Moreover, they can impede the proper functioning of the liver, stomach, and pancreas, leading to a range of disorders including gastritis, gastroparesis, irritable bowel syndrome (IBS), diabetes, and chronic fatigue.

When patients are unaware of these subluxations and experience only the physical symptoms associated with them, they may embark on a journey of trying various medications, herbs, supplements, and even suspect infections or nutritional deficiencies. They might resort to antidepressants, stimulants, or different diets in their quest for relief. However, what they may not realize is that their underlying issue is mechanical in nature. To address it effectively, they should consider a chiropractic perspective that focuses on the mechanical aspects of their condition.

Remarkably, chiropractic doctors have, in some instances, achieved remarkable results in treating conditions such as blindness by addressing nerve compression in the neck. They have successfully alleviated IBS symptoms by adjusting thoracic and dorsal vertebrae.

Post-traumatic stress disorder has been improved by correcting neck posture. Even conditions like hiatal hernias have seen improvement through the correction of subluxations and the relief of nerves that control the diaphragm.

Dr. Suzuki Kuny, in his book "Health Revolution," shared his personal journey of overcoming epilepsy. By a stroke of luck, he stumbled upon a surprising revelation: the trigger for his epilepsy was a misaligned coccyx, a critical part of the spine.

Through the correction of his coccyx alignment, he not only managed to heal from epilepsy but also freed himself from the reliance on numerous ineffective medications prescribed by his healthcare providers. These medications had not only failed to alleviate his condition but had also contributed to the development of iatrogenic ailments, including gastrointestinal issues and pain.

Dr. Kuny emphasized that through spinal and coccyx adjustments, he experienced a complete recovery, and he felt compelled to share his remarkable testimonial in his book for the benefit of others.

Within the pages of this book, we will explore a selection of exercises that are both time-efficient and adaptable for anyone, anywhere. These exercises have the potential to invigorate and align your spine effectively.
Some of these exercises require no special equipment and can be performed independently, while others may necessitate the assistance of a device, making them accessible even for individuals with health challenges.

The underlying concept and rationale behind these exercises are rooted in the desire to transport your spine back to a state of relaxation, free from the burdens and subluxations that may have accumulated over time.

The aim is to restore your spine to the vibrant, flexible, and well-aligned condition it once enjoyed.

<u>THE EXERCISES</u>

The Gold fish exercise:

The Goldfish exercise, credited to its inventor Katsuzo Nishi and a vital component of his six health laws, serves the purpose of spinal adjustment and subluxation correction. Its name, the "Goldfish exercise," is derived from the resemblance of the human body's movements during the exercise to those of a swimming goldfish.

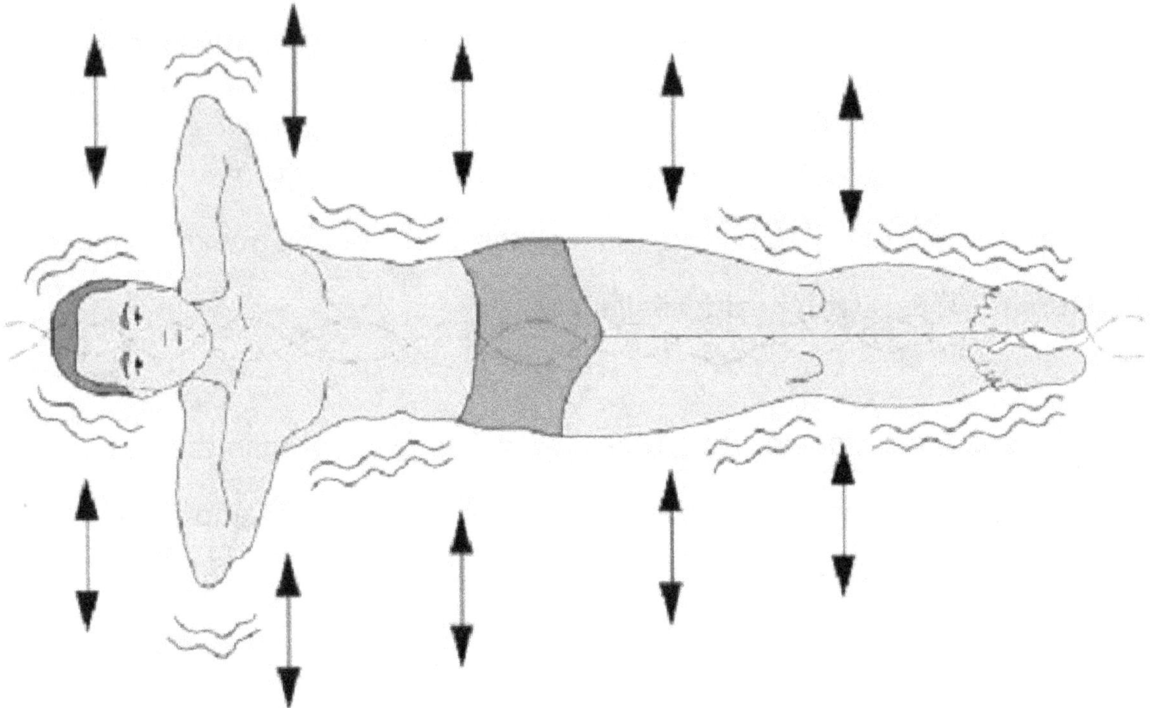

As previously explained, our nerves extend from the left and right sides of the spinal column. During the performance of this exercise, each time the spine bends to the right, it results in increased freedom and stronger nervous impulses on the left side. Conversely, when the spine bends to the left, it widens the foramens (openings) on the right side between the vertebrae, freeing the nerves and enhancing impulse strength on that side. By swaying alternately to the left and right, nerve impulses become increasingly pronounced in both directions. It's akin to an electric impulse emanating from the spinal center and spreading outwards to both the left and right sides.

This phenomenon leads to the constriction of capillaries throughout the body while the exercise is in progress. Additionally, it encourages a balanced distribution of nerve impulses throughout the body, promoting symmetry in innervation.

The exercise also facilitates the return of blood from the legs to the heart, benefiting blood circulation and the cardiovascular system. Furthermore, it aids in the movement of lymph, helping to alleviate stagnant edemas.

Upon concluding the exercise, a tingling sensation is often experienced throughout the body. This sensation is attributed to the dilation of previously constricted capillaries.

The oscillation of the spine not only corrects subluxations but also contributes to the repositioning of many body organs. As a result, this exercise proves highly beneficial for conditions like gastroptosis, where organs have shifted from their normal positions.

To begin, lie down flat on your back. Then, gently flex your toes towards your knees, forming an acute angle, while ensuring both soles remain even. Place your hands crossed against the fourth or tit cervical vertebra (near the neck). Maintaining this posture, create a swaying motion akin to that of a swimming goldfish. Dedicate one to two minutes to practice this exercise every morning and evening.

After addressing outward and inward subluxations of the vertebrae using a flat bed and ensuring the physiological curvature of the cervical vertebrae with a solid pillow, it's time to target scoliosis (lateral subluxation) with the goldfish exercise.

This particular exercise aids in rectifying the misalignment of vertebral outlets through which spinal nerves emerge. This correction alleviates undue pressure on these nerves and mitigates peripheral nerve paralysis. Consequently, it contributes to improving the overall nervous system function and regulating blood circulation.

Furthermore, this exercise promotes regular bowel movement, reducing the risk of intestinal torsion or obstruction. This, in turn, supports the physiological functioning of the intestines.

Additionally, it helps in harmonizing the imbalances between the left and right sides of the body caused by professional movements, sports, and other activities. Over time, it fosters a harmonious equilibrium between body and mind.

To perform the goldfish exercise effectively, complete relaxation is essential. Alternatively, one can hold on to a pair of tall crutches and gently sway the hips from side to side to eliminate spinal distortions before attempting the standard goldfish exercise. When applying this exercise to a patient, an assistant can hold the patient's ankles and gently shake them laterally to achieve the desired effect.

For individuals who may find the Goldfish exercise challenging, there exists a helpful device known as the Chi Machine. This device is remarkably straightforward to use, featuring a design that includes handles for each ankle and the ability to oscillate the body gently from left to right.

To utilize the Chi Machine, all that is required is to recline on your back, place your ankles securely in the ankle holders, and activate the machine. There are several variations of Chi machines available, all operating on the same fundamental principle.

However, some models provide additional features such as speed control, which proves particularly beneficial for elderly or unwell individuals who may need to adjust the oscillation speed. Additionally, certain machines come equipped with timers, allowing you to set a specific duration for the machine to carry out its gentle body oscillations.

The Chi Machine offers a profoundly relaxing and rejuvenating experience, effectively combating fatigue. It revitalizes the body and assists in achieving a more upright posture.

The Mid Position

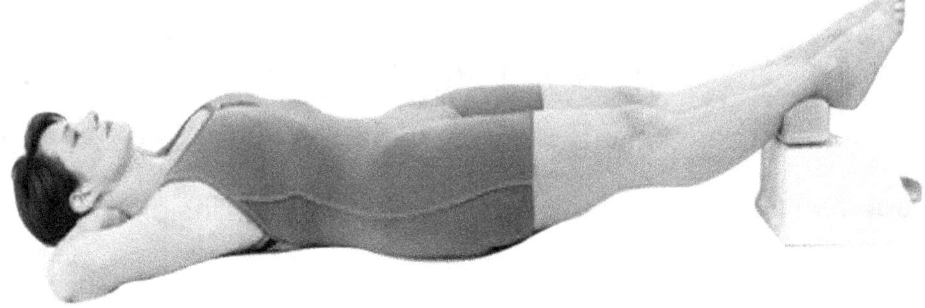

The Goldfish Position

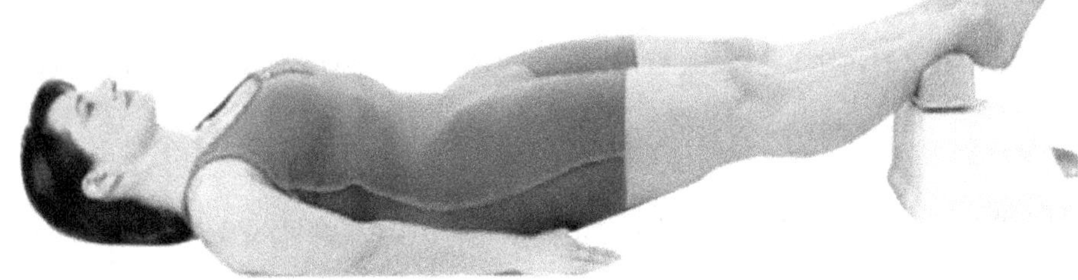

The Stretched Back Position

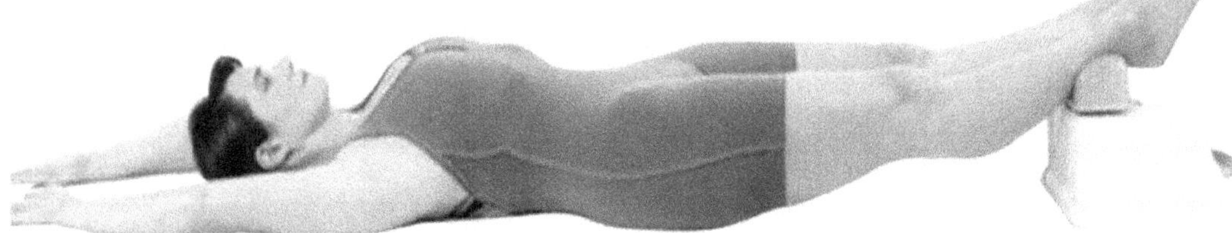

The Second Exercise

Sleeping on your back on a hard bed:

"l'ami de la colonne faible est le plan dur, table ou lit a matelas mince sur planches." Dr. Andre de Sambucy, Gymnastique corrective et traitement respiratoire, page 120.
" The best friend of the weak spine is a hard flat bed" Dr. Andre de Sambyc, Corrective gymnastic and respiratory therapy.

Another valuable tool for spinal adjustment isn't an exercise but rather a specific sleeping posture. Sleeping on your back can effectively align the spinal column as the firm surface of the bed exerts pressure on the spinous processes, promoting the perfect alignment of the entire thoracic and lumbar vertebrae. This alignment not only has a positive impact on spinal health but also enhances the efficiency of the liver.

Individuals who adopt the habit of sleeping on their back often wake up feeling refreshed and invigorated in the morning, thanks to the liver's improved functionality. This posture allows the body's organs to assume their natural positions without exerting pressure on one another. In contrast, sleeping on the left side can lead to the liver pressing against the heart, stomach, pancreas, and lungs, potentially causing breathing difficulties. On the right side, the liver faces pressure from the heart and stomach.

Sleeping on one's back also aids in the venous return process, facilitating the return of blood to the heart. Moreover, this sleeping position, particularly on a firm surface like a hard floor, can help address lumbar subluxations, promoting the effective functioning of the kidneys, sexual organs, and lower limbs. Remarkably, this method of sleeping has the potential to provide rapid relief from sciatic nerve pain.

According to Katsuzo Nishi, sleeping on a hard floor enhances the immune system by ensuring that nerves and blood vessels are evenly distributed across the sleeping surface. This, in turn, stimulates the production of life ions in the body, fostering increased vitality.

In his book " the Nishi Health engineering" about the flat bad, Nishi mentioned that Among the various vertebrae in the spine, certain positions are particularly susceptible to unfavorable subluxations. The first and fourth cervical vertebrae are notably vulnerable to subluxation. If subluxation occurs in the first cervical vertebra, it can have a significant impact on various parts of the body, including the eyes, face, neck, lungs, diaphragm, stomach, kidneys, suprarenal gland, heart, spleen, and intestines. On the other hand, subluxation in the fourth cervical vertebra is more likely to affect the eyes, face, neck, lungs, diaphragm, liver, heart, spleen, suprarenal gland, nose, heart, teeth, throat, and more.

Within the thoracic vertebrae, the second, fifth, and tenth vertebrae are particularly prone to subluxation. Subluxation of the second thoracic vertebra can impact the lungs and pleura. If it occurs in the fifth thoracic vertebra, potential issues may arise in the eyes, throat, stomach, and thyroid gland. Subluxation of the tenth thoracic vertebra may lead to disorders in the eyes, heart, kidneys, intestines, nose, and more.

Moving to the lumbar vertebrae, the second and fifth vertebrae are predisposed to subluxation. Subluxation of the second lumbar vertebra may manifest as conditions like bladder inflammation, appendicitis, and sexual organ-related concerns. In the case of subluxation in the fifth lumbar vertebra, it might be associated with issues in the anus, possibly leading to conditions like hemorrhoids.

While the mentioned vertebrae are particularly prone to subluxation from a dynamic perspective, it's important to note that external factors, occupational demands, injuries, or other causes can lead to subluxation in any of the vertebrae. Consequently, a wide range of diseases or disorders can be attributed to spinal column misalignment. Conversely, even minor disorders in internal organs can result in undesirable conditions within the spinal column.

In her book "The Key to Rejuvenation," Mary Ellison reveals that the key to rejuvenating her body and facial appearance was a simple practice: sleeping on her back on a firm surface, such as a hard floor.

If you suffer from acid reflux, you can elevate your bed slightly around the head while sleeping on your back on a hard floor. Some people for some reason, they can get their acid reflux aggravated when they sleep on their back. So elevating their bed from the side of the head can help with this issue.

THE THIRD TOOL

The Cervical Traction Device:

The neck is an important link between the rest of body and head. It is neurological link. A circulatioary bridge and pillar that holds the hed above the body.

It appears that the subluxation of neck vertebrae may be a root cause of numerous diseases.

A neck massage by the Danish Osteopath Stanley Rosenberg was enough to heal an autistic kid form his autism. Yes. You got this right.

Could dysfunction in the medulla oblongata be a potential factor contributing to autism? Dr Stanley Rosenberg claims to have successfully treated an American child with autism using neck massage techniques, as shown in the video below.

Dr. Ali Musaraf, an Indian-born physician practicing in the UK, explores the significance of neck health in his book "The Neck Connection." He emphasizes the delicate nature of blood delivery in the neck and how any disruption in blood supply, leading to insufficient glucose and oxygen, can impact the medulla oblongata. He suggests that simple neck massage techniques can help restore proper blood flow and potentially alleviate various health issues.

Dr. Bodo Kuklinski, a German biohacker with a focus on mitochondria, shares a similar perspective. He asserts that neck circulation plays a crucial role in the optimal functioning of the medulla oblongata and goes as far as claiming that neck massage therapy can contribute to the restoration of mitochondrial function. His book, "Your Neck – the 'Weakest Link': Causes, Effects, and Successful Therapy," delves into these ideas.

These discussions draw parallels to the renowned Spanish doctor, Asuero, known for his remarkable treatments that were often viewed as miraculous. Some individuals who were wheelchair-bound reportedly regained the ability to walk after undergoing Asuero's galvanic current nasal therapy, which aimed to restore the function of the medulla oblongata.

In summary, various experts and practitioners suggest that addressing neck health and circulation through massage techniques could potentially have far-reaching therapeutic benefits, including the restoration of medulla oblongata function and the mitigation of certain health conditions.

A cervical traction device is a medical apparatus designed to provide traction or decompression to the cervical spine, which is the region of the spine located in the neck. These devices are used in medical settings for therapeutic purposes and can also be prescribed for home use in some cases.

The main goal of cervical traction is to relieve pressure on the cervical vertebrae, discs, and surrounding structures, such as nerves and soft tissues. This can be beneficial for various medical conditions and symptoms, including:

A cervical traction device is a medical apparatus designed to provide traction or decompression to the cervical spine, which is the region of the spine located in the neck. These devices are used in medical settings for therapeutic purposes and can also be prescribed for home use in some cases.

The main goal of cervical traction is to relieve pressure on the cervical vertebrae, discs, and surrounding structures, such as nerves and soft tissues.

This can be beneficial for various medical conditions and symptoms, including:

Neck pain: Cervical traction can help alleviate neck pain caused by conditions like cervical disc herniation, cervical stenosis, or muscle spasms.

<u>Nerve compression</u>: If a nerve in the cervical spine is compressed or pinched, traction can help reduce the pressure and alleviate symptoms like radiating pain, numbness, or tingling into the arms and hands.

<u>Cervical radiculopathy</u>: This condition involves the irritation or compression of nerve roots in the cervical spine, often resulting in arm pain or weakness. Cervical traction may provide relief.

<u>Cervical spondylosis</u>: Also known as cervical osteoarthritis, this condition involves degeneration of the cervical vertebrae and discs. Traction can help manage pain and improve mobility.

<u>Muscle tension and spasms</u>: Cervical traction can help relax neck muscles and reduce muscle spasms.

Cervical traction can be administered using various methods, including manual traction performed by a healthcare provider, mechanical devices, or over-the-door traction units. Home cervical traction devices are designed for self-administration under the guidance of a healthcare professional.

These devices typically involve a harness or collar that wraps around the neck and is connected to a weight, air pressure, or mechanical system that gently pulls on the neck, creating a stretching or decompressive force. The duration and intensity of cervical traction are determined by the patient's condition and healthcare provider's recommendations.

A cervical traction device is a medical apparatus designed to provide traction or decompression to the cervical spine, which is the region of the spine located in the neck. These devices are used in medical settings for therapeutic purposes and can also be prescribed for home use in some cases.

The main goal of cervical traction is to relieve pressure on the cervical vertebrae, discs, and surrounding structures, such as nerves and soft tissues.

This can be beneficial for various medical conditions and symptoms, including:

<u>Neck pain</u>: Cervical traction can help alleviate neck pain caused by conditions like cervical disc herniation, cervical stenosis, or muscle spasms.

<u>Nerve compression</u>: If a nerve in the cervical spine is compressed or pinched, traction can help reduce the pressure and alleviate symptoms like radiating pain, numbness, or tingling into the arms and hands.

<u>Cervical radiculopathy</u>: This condition involves the irritation or compression of nerve roots in the cervical spine, often resulting in arm pain or weakness. Cervical traction may provide relief.

<u>Cervical spondylosis</u>: Also known as cervical osteoarthritis, this condition involves degeneration of the cervical vertebrae and discs. Traction can help manage pain and improve mobility.

<u>Muscle tension and spasms</u>: Cervical traction can help relax neck muscles and reduce muscle spasms.

Cervical traction can be administered using various methods, including manual traction performed by a healthcare provider, mechanical devices, or over-the-door traction units. Home cervical traction devices are designed for self-administration under the guidance of a healthcare professional.

These devices typically involve a harness or collar that wraps around the neck and is connected to a weight, air pressure, or mechanical system that gently pulls on the neck, creating a stretching or decompressive force. The duration and intensity of cervical traction are determined by the patient's condition and healthcare provider's recommendations.

Among the safer options for cervical traction devices are those that can be conveniently set up using a door. Known as over-the-door cervical traction devices, these are suitable for use both in therapy offices and at home.

This type of traction typically involves securing a harness or cushioned sling around the head and neck. The harness is then connected to a system consisting of a rope and pulley, which is positioned over a door.

In some cases, an additional weight may be attached to the end of the rope, or you can manually pull the rope to create the stretching effect on the neck.

Neck traction therapy should ideally be performed at least twice a day, with each session lasting for approximately 5 to 10 minutes.

When engaging in neck traction, it's crucial to exercise caution and avoid excessive force.

The goal is to gently guide your head and assist your cervical vertebrae in the process of readjustment and realignment.

Consistency is key, and it's essential not to overextend or pull excessively.

The primary objective is to promote healing within your body rather than causing harm or injury.

The Fourth Tool

The Wooden Pillow

The wooden pillow, a unique and innovative tool, plays a pivotal role in addressing cervical subluxation. Unlike traditional traction devices that rely on pulling forces, the wooden pillow takes a different approach. It does not tug at the head and neck but instead exerts a gentle yet purposeful pressure against the cervical vertebrae, aiding in the restoration of the spine's natural curved and concave curvature.

In our modern lives, characterized by prolonged hours spent in sedentary positions and often straining neck postures, this natural neck curvature can become compromised. The wooden pillow steps in as a remedy, helping individuals regain this essential alignment. However, it's important to note that the initial experience with a wooden pillow may not always be entirely comfortable.

When you first rest your neck and head upon the wooden pillow, you might encounter a sensation of discomfort or mild discomfort. This sensation, paradoxically, serves as a kind of barometer for your health. It signals that your neck was not previously perfectly aligned, and the discomfort is a sign that the wooden pillow is beginning to address and rectify the issue.

Ideally, the goal is to gradually transition into sleeping on the wooden pillow for the entire night. This extended duration of use allows the wooden pillow to exert its corrective influence effectively. However, it's understandable that many people are not accustomed to the firmness of a wooden pillow initially. As a result, a gradual approach may be more comfortable.

In the beginning, you can start by using the wooden pillow for shorter periods, perhaps just 10 to 15 minutes at a time. This short-term usage serves as an introductory phase, enabling your body to adapt to the unique support provided by the wooden pillow. Over time, as your comfort level increases and your body adjusts, you can extend the duration of use, eventually progressing to sleeping on it throughout the night.

The wooden pillow's design and function are rooted in the understanding that the neck's alignment profoundly influences overall spinal health. By applying gentle pressure to the cervical vertebrae, this pillow promotes the restoration of the neck's natural curve, which can be compromised by our modern lifestyles and habits.

The benefits of using a wooden pillow extend beyond mere posture correction. As the cervical vertebrae gradually realign, individuals may experience improvements in various aspects of their well-being. Many users report reduced neck and back pain, enhanced sleep quality, and a sense of increased vitality and energy.

It's worth noting that while the wooden pillow may initially feel unfamiliar, its transformative potential for neck health and overall wellness can be truly remarkable. As you embark on this journey of spinal realignment, remember to be patient with yourself and allow your body the time it needs to adapt. The discomfort you may initially encounter is a positive sign of progress, signaling the positive changes occurring within your body.

In conclusion, the wooden pillow offers a unique and natural solution for addressing cervical subluxation and restoring the neck's essential curvature. Its gentle pressure and support can lead to improvements in posture, reduced pain, and enhanced overall well-being. While the transition to sleeping on a wooden pillow may require some patience and gradual adjustment, the potential benefits for your health and vitality make it a valuable investment in your well-being.

As per Katsuzo Nishi's teachings, the wooden pillow not only contributes to the overall well-being of the vagus nerve but also offers therapeutic benefits for oral and thyroid health. Additionally, it can potentially assist in dental adjustments within the jaws.

The Fifth Tool:

The Inversion Table

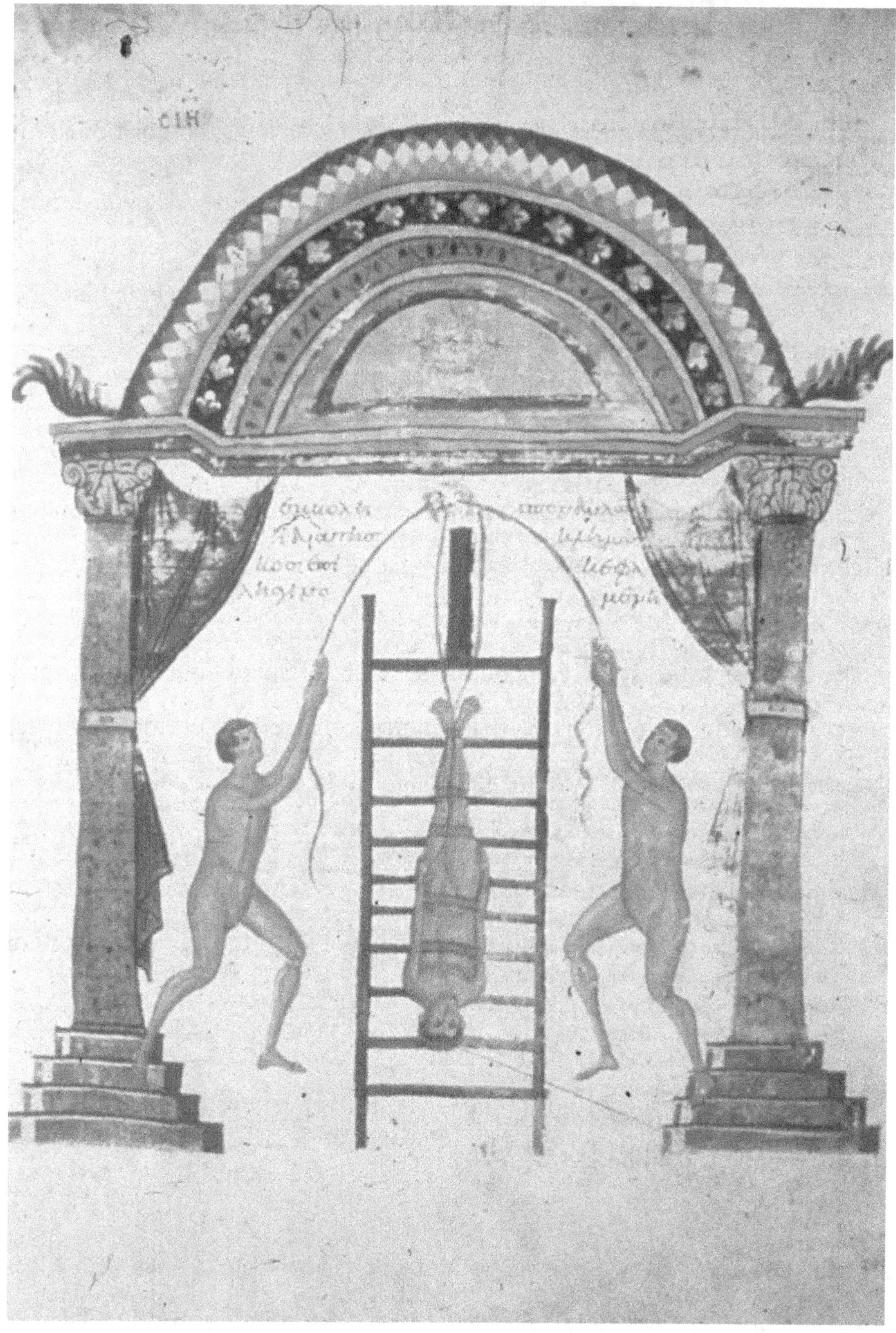

The inversion table offers a contrasting approach to the traditional neck traction device. With this apparatus, the body is suspended upside down. Inversion tables are specially designed devices that enable an individual to recline into an inverted position at adjustable angles.

The user typically lies on a platform, while their ankles are securely held in place by a bracket equipped with a ratcheting mechanism.

The inversion table operates on the principle of utilizing gravity to its advantage. When a person reclines on this table, their body weight naturally exerts a downward pull on the spine, effectively relieving subluxations and correcting vertebral misalignments.

Additionally, this gravitational force encourages increased blood flow towards the brain, enhancing oxygenation to this vital organ. Furthermore, inversion promotes the activity of the parasympathetic nervous system, fostering a state of relaxation.

The inversion table's benefits extend to the entire spine, spanning from the neck through the thoracic and lumbar regions. It achieves this by gently stretching these segments of the spinal column.

Moreover, this inversion process aids in the facilitation of venous blood return to the heart, capitalizing on the influence of gravity.

For those who are new to using an inversion table, it is advisable to start with a less steep angle of incline for a brief duration, typically around 1 to 2 minutes. Gradually, as one becomes more accustomed to the sensation and effects, they can increase the angle to achieve a complete inversion and comfortably remain in this position for a duration of 10 to 15 minutes.

THE LAST METHOD IN OUR SELF CHIROPRACTIC IS THE HIDA BREATHING METHOD:

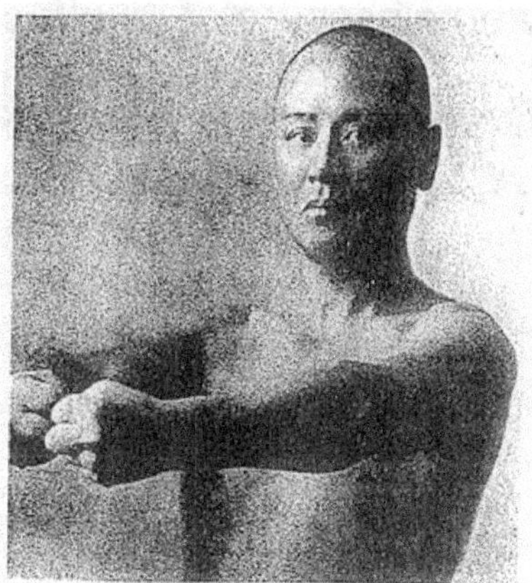

The Hida breathing method encompasses both a specialized breathing technique and a posture correction method.

It entails lying on a firm surface, typically on your back, while practicing diaphragmatic breathing.

This approach serves a dual purpose by addressing both breathing patterns and actively aligning the body's posture.

In essence, Hida breathing aims to realign the center of gravity to its natural position, restoring balance to the entire body.

Hypermobility and the loss of the center of gravity:

The loss of center of gravity is the cause of most diseases. Actually, NASA can pay you 20 000 dollars for one year if you sleep upside down so scientists can study effect of antigravity on human health. When we lose the center of gravity, we lose balance.

The inclined bed therapy helps people because of its effect on the center of gravity and circulation. Its inventor Andrew Fletcher claims that the height of people will increase by up to 1 inch by doing IBD.

You can see now that only Osteopaths study this subject seriously.
The French mechanical engineer and inventor Gorgia Knap who allegedly invented the first motorcycle wrote a book about the importance of the center of gravity in health and disease and that its loss is the cause of all diseases. He invented a set o exercises to do to correct and restore a normal or close to perfect center of gravity.

The Israeli inventor and physicist Moshe Feldenkrais also had the same theory as Kap and he invented his own method of correcting the posture and bringing the center of gravity back to normal.

Most Animals know that by their natural instincts. Most of you have seen dogs or cats or horses shaking their bodies fast by a quick swing movement along the column vertebrae to bring back to normalcy the center of gravity.
And this is not a new science, ancient doctors like Avicenna or Hippocrates knew about it and wrote books showing the methods they used to correct the posture, the spine and the center of gravity.

Maybe the loss of the center of gravity in Mars what made Elon Musk say that he believes that the first human colony in the red planet will die quickly. Because Astronauts all of them suffer from the effect of the loss of gravity. And maybe living in higher towers is not good for health as well.

Harumitsu Hida

Let's delve into the breathing technique attributed to, but before we dive into the method itself, let's provide a brief introduction to him.

Harumitsu Hida was born on December 25, 1883. His father, Tatemitsu Kawai, was a physician. When he was six years old, his mother and three of his siblings died from illness, and he himself was very frail and sickly.

Here is how he describes himself in his writings:

"I was the eighth child of a family living in dim circumstances. My father was already 50 years old at my birth, and my mother, being older, lacked sufficient breast milk. I was very thin, with a face and gait resembling that of a girl. When playing, other children would often carry me on their backs because I was so light. Guests in our home would frequently inquire if I were a girl. My bones were slender, and my skin was pale, dry, and lacking in any fat. This is why I was frequently rubbed with oil all over my body...

This was how death seemed to be approaching me, just as it had taken my brothers and sisters. When I was six years old, I contracted typhus, which led to pneumonia and asthma accompanied by severe diarrhea. With a fever of 40 degrees, I was so weakened that doctors declared my case to be hopeless.

My father, who had lost a son in the same year, was on the verge of despair. The Day of the Dead was approaching. He said, 'I wish for him to survive, even if it's just for these three days, so we can spend the Day of the Dead together.' I did not die, but I was literally skin and bones...

I remained continuously ill throughout my childhood and became familiar with all sorts of medications. My digestive system was fragile, I constantly suffered from migraines and dizziness, and I caught colds all the time. The scope of my life was confined to a sickbed. The image of my childhood is that of a boy with skin and bones, standing sadly, shrinking his miserable body in the cold wind. What a dark childhood it was!...

Later, my classmates nicknamed me 'reed leaf,' and I was unable to revolt against such a humiliating nickname. I simply had to accept it, and when it became too painful, I would slip away unnoticed... My biceps were no thicker than my wrists, and I was ashamed of my body. I sighed, thinking that my body couldn't handle the slightest effort. I was indeed a 'reed leaf'..."

He Decides to Transform Himself :

At eighteen, the awareness of his desperate fragility led him to make the decision to transform his own body.

"One day, I began to contemplate my future, my social destiny. I became afraid and started self-criticism. I said to myself, 'Hey, Harumitsu, what are you going to do when you're so worthless? A little cold, and you're already catching a cold. You eat a bit, and you have a stomachache, followed by diarrhea. You walk a bit, and you're tired. When you sleep, you only have nightmares. What's the point of living like this? What a sad life you lead; the only thing you're good for is to feed the earth of your grave. '

This dreadful thought passed through my heart, and a great whirlwind rose within my chest, oppressed by a sense of inferiority... Deep down, I wanted to attain good health and a robust body, like a thirsty person desires a drink. I didn't just want good health to avoid illness; I wanted to become strong, truly strong, so that I could courageously do something for others. This desire was a determination in which I invested my entire being, ultimately allowing me to transform my body and mind. It was in April of the year 1900; I was 17 years old...

Plants grow like flames in the summer, then autumn arrives, followed by winter, and they retreat beneath the snow. However, they rejoice in the sun's return when spring arrives. But if heavy snow were to cover these plants for four or five years, they would all die. Isn't my body similar to these plants, covered by snow for too long to be able to revive in spring? Hasn't my vitality completely withered away? In such a state, if I were to exercise, I risked destroying myself completely. What should I do then? Well, I simply have to die...

In my state, there were only two options: either I win or I die. It is a person's honor to die while striving to achieve their goal. That's how I took the first step...

I believed that I needed to establish a solid foundation for my endeavor. I had to understand the human body's structure. To do that, I gathered anatomy and physiology books from my father's library. I immersed myself in reading these books with respect, much like a Christian reads the Bible because they were decisive works for my existence in this world...

Studying the body's internal functions, organs, and viscera deeply struck me with the mystery of life in nature. With surprise and profound admiration, I had to acknowledge divine creation and developed the conviction that there is a close connection between belief and science. Learning about metabolism and cell renewal particularly encouraged me. The human body is not like a stone or rubber statue; it functions actively and is capable of self-renewal. If healthy people's cells renew themselves every seven years, I would take ten years to escape my state of weakness. I would take fifteen years to reach an ordinary body. By persevering for twenty years, investing my life in it, I believed I could surpass the ordinary level. In spring, a plum tree will bloom even more fragrantly if it has endured a harsher winter. The emotion of this decision brought tears to my eyes... When I read the phrase, 'An exquisite scent of spring plum blossoms forms precisely because it has endured the severity of winter under the snow,' I was moved to tears. I needed patience and sustained effort! My path is undoubtedly long and difficult. I must become like a plum blossom. Patience and effort!"

Solitary Study :

"Following my readings on anatomy and physiology, I collected all sorts of books on physical exercises, as well as medical, hygiene, and sports physiology books. Every time I encountered a new exercise, I would immediately practice it and contemplate it. The abundance of practices compelled me to make choices. I should mention that I never sought a personal method; I was solely looking for a way to save myself from my physical misery...

So, I took a perfect body as my model: the bone structure, muscles, shape, internal organs, and athletic capacity. In a way, it was ridiculous for someone as wretched as me to take the ideal body as a model... Therefore, I didn't stop at common methods that aimed at trivial effectiveness, such as simple gymnastics, deep breathing, cold-water ablutions, and a few hygiene methods aimed at minor well-being. My goal was to enhance the quality and effectiveness of all these exercises through a systematic approach...

I sought a method that fulfilled the following conditions:

- The method's practice must be active rather than passive since the aim was to attain a strong and powerful body.

- The exercise must be an end in itself and not merely a preparation for a technique.

- The exercise should not require spending money or the use of equipment. Health should be achieved through the body's sole effort.

- Most importantly, the exercise should not demand a significant amount of time. If the exercise was lengthy, it would become difficult to perform daily and could lead to unnecessary fatigue.

And so, I built my decision to embark on this path of body transformation, and whenever I heard of someone who had deeply invested themselves to achieve their goal, I sincerely studied their approach. How many times was I encouraged by others when I almost gave up? Because I had no certainty of success in my endeavor, but I had to continue regardless of the pain of failure...

When I read the translation of the novel 'Monte Cristo' (by Alexandre Dumas), I was profoundly moved by a prisoner who had spent seven years digging a tunnel and then had to start over because he had dug in the wrong direction... I would take ten years to have a body capable of escaping illness, and after fifteen years, I would have a normal body. I will succeed, I will succeed... A prisoner strives to succeed in their prison; I, at least, am in a free world. How could I not try?

Every time I asked my father for a new book, he bought it for me without asking about my goal. He was simply happy to see me studious. At home, during my abdominal and muscle strengthening exercises, I fell, hitting the floor with my feet and hands, tearing the tatami mats in several places, dislodging floor supports, breaking or puncturing sliding doors, yet my father never scolded me. On the contrary, he seemed delighted to see me, who had always been so sick, moving with such vigor today. Did he let me do it out of love and pity for a motherless child? My father, like my older brother, let me do whatever I wanted. Despite my fragility, it was thanks to their love that I could continue building my path. Every time I recall my father's affection, it brings tears to my eyes..."

First Achievement

"Nothing is as extraordinary as an act performed with vital determination; ultimate sincerity can touch the heavens. I succeeded in reaching my first goal.

Because my health improved rapidly. The color of my skin changed. My arms, which were as thin as sticks, became adorned with imposing muscles, and my shoulders became broad. I felt great in my own skin! My face reflected vitality; my eyes were alive, my nose and mouth were taut and full of strength. Where was the shadow of the sickly child of the past? Yet, only two years had passed since I began, thinking it would take more than ten years to achieve an ordinary body..."

Following our brief introduction to Harumitsu Hida, let's delve into his potent breathing technique, known as the "Normal Posture Breathing Method." This method is refreshingly straightforward, albeit it requires you to assume a supine position on a rigid floor. The purpose of this choice is to facilitate the correction of spinal alignment.
In this reclined position, you initiate the practice with a deliberate inhalation, emphasizing the expansion of the abdomen and activation of the diaphragm. Upon exhalation, you allow the belly to naturally deflate.

It's crucial to maintain a steady pace, with each inhalation lasting a minimum of 4 seconds and each exhalation taking about 5 to 6 seconds.
This routine is ideally practiced for a duration of 10 to 20 minutes, either once or twice a day.

The benefits of this potent technique are manifold: it significantly enhances lung capacity and stands as an excellent exercise for refreshing our lung function.

Moreover, this method serves as a reset for the autonomic nervous system, boosts immunity, aligns the spine, aids digestion, and promotes mental clarity. In essence, this exercise forms the cornerstone of the Hida Health Method.